A TO Z

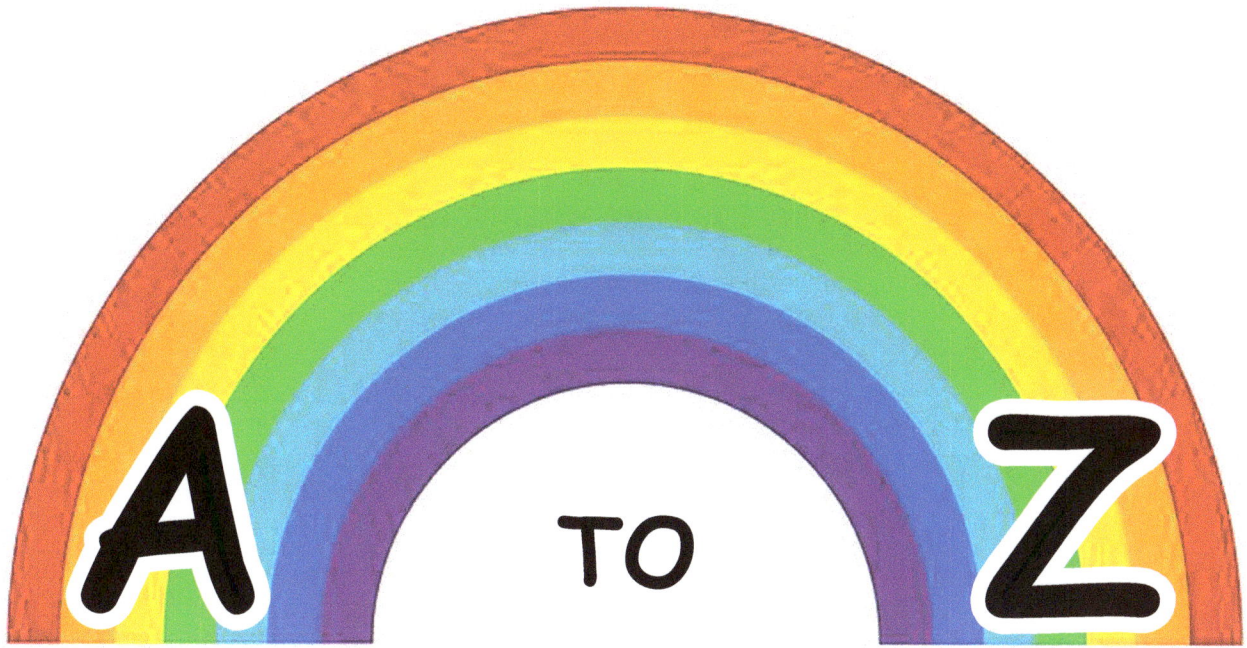

SPEECH THERAPY

Written by
Penelope Hope

Illustrated by
Shea Peters

Waldenhouse Publishers, Inc.
Walden, Tennessee

A TO Z: SPEECH THERAPY

Illustrated by Shea Peters
Published by Waldenhouse Publishers, Inc.
100 Clegg Street, Signal Mountain, Tennessee 37377 USA
423-886-2721   www.waldenhouse.com

ISBN: 978-1-94758-958-2
Library of Congress Control Number: 2021943081
Each letter of the alphabet is repeated in alliterative words printed in large, easy to read type on a single page. Every letter and text block is accompanied by an active illustration of the letter sound. Repetition of letter sounds help with speech. Suitable for children and adult English speakers.
-- Provided by publisher

HEA035000 HEALTH & FITNESS / Hearing & Speech
EDU029080 EDUCATION / Teaching Methods & Materials / Language Arts
LAN018000 LANGUAGE ARTS & DISCIPLINES / Speech & Pronunciation

Preface

Using the letters of the Alphabet my thought is to write sentences with six words in each sentence starting with that specific letter explaining the picture above it. This allows repetition of the sound of the letters helping readers with speech. There are also extra items in some of the pictures that actually use that letter written. Repeating the sound of the letter helps with a person's speech.

Dedicated to

My Aunt Runa Johnson
in Memoriam.

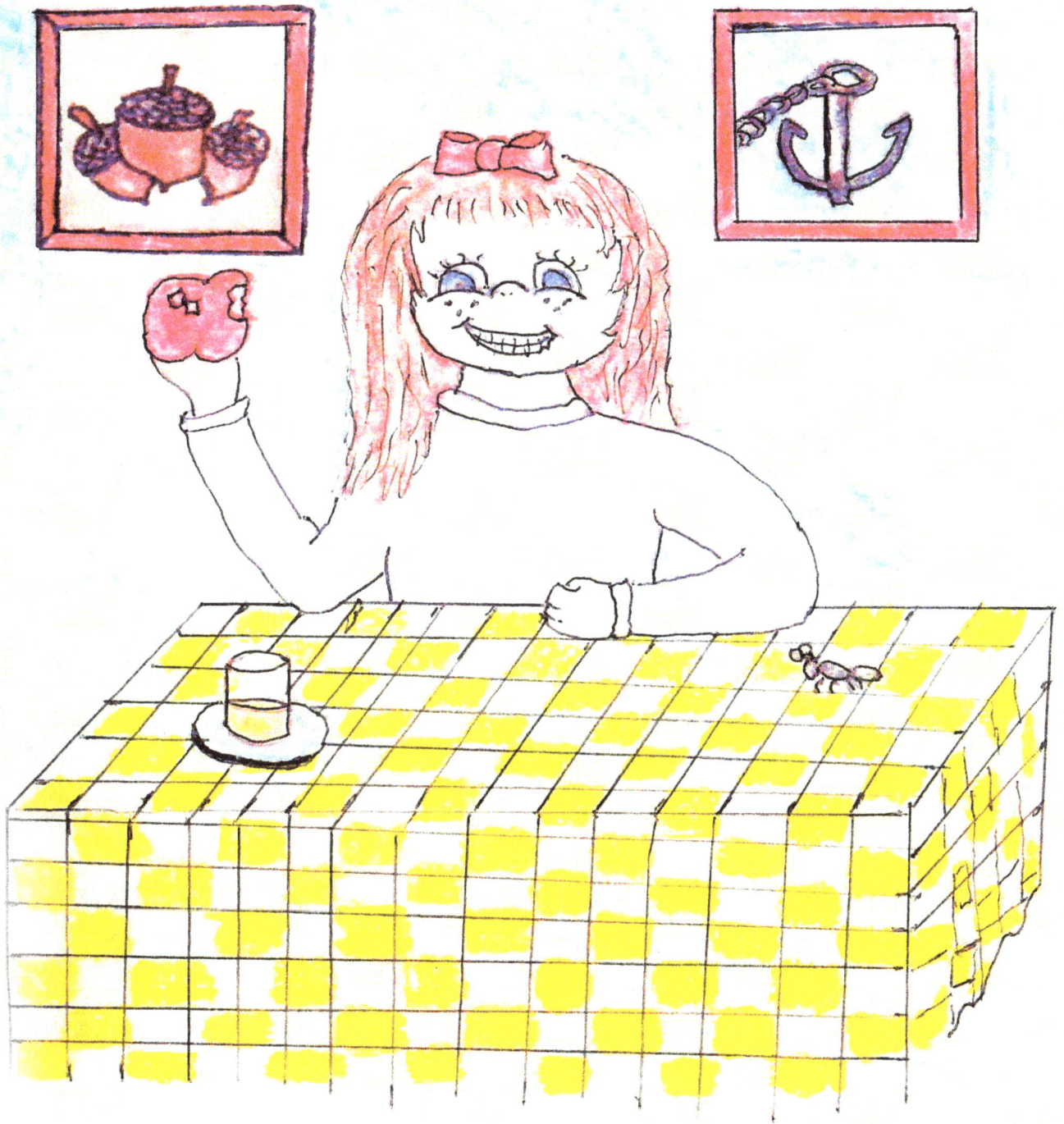

Aa Alice ate an apple and enjoyed
all she ate.

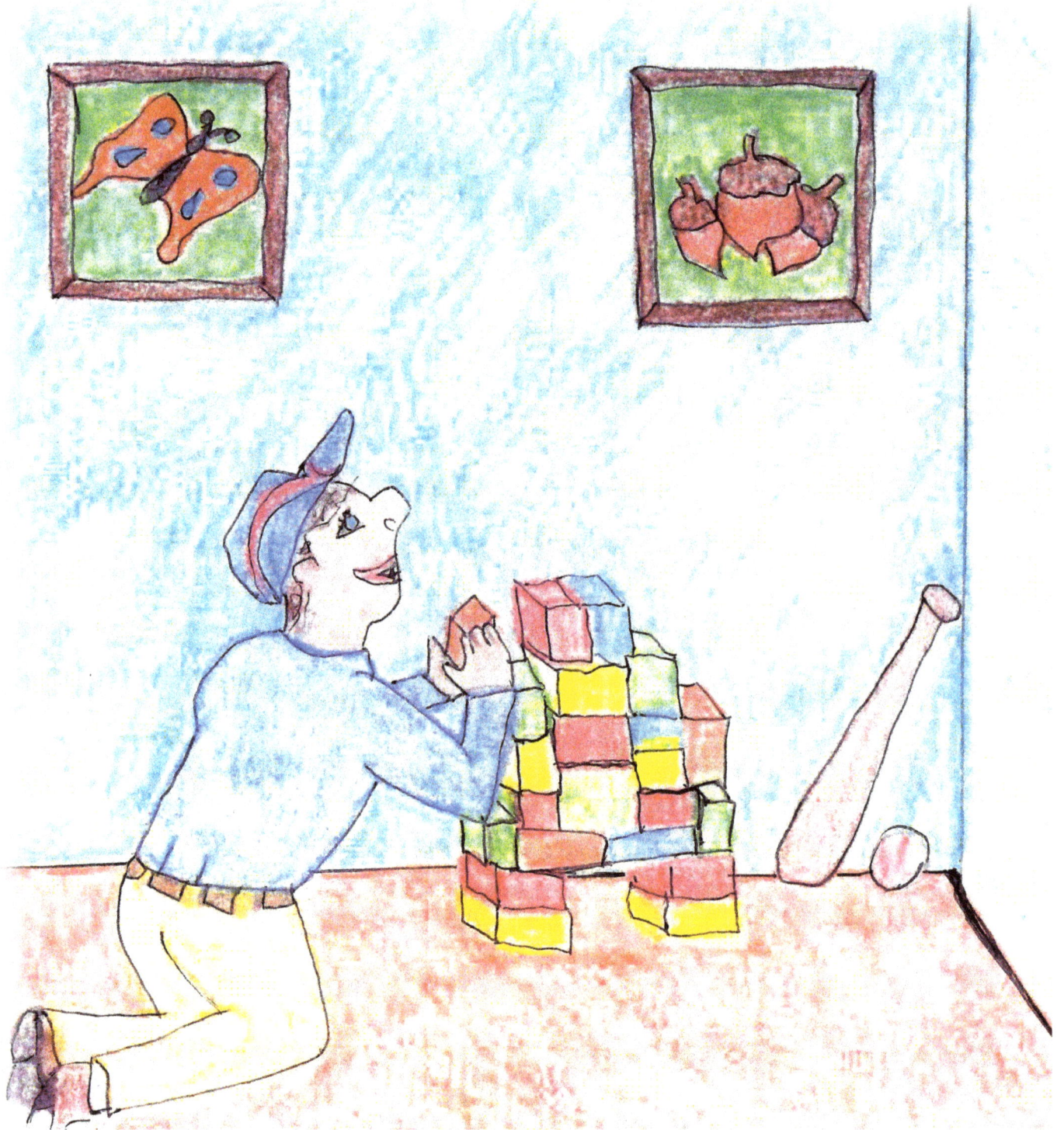

Bb Bobby builds big buildings with bunches of blocks.

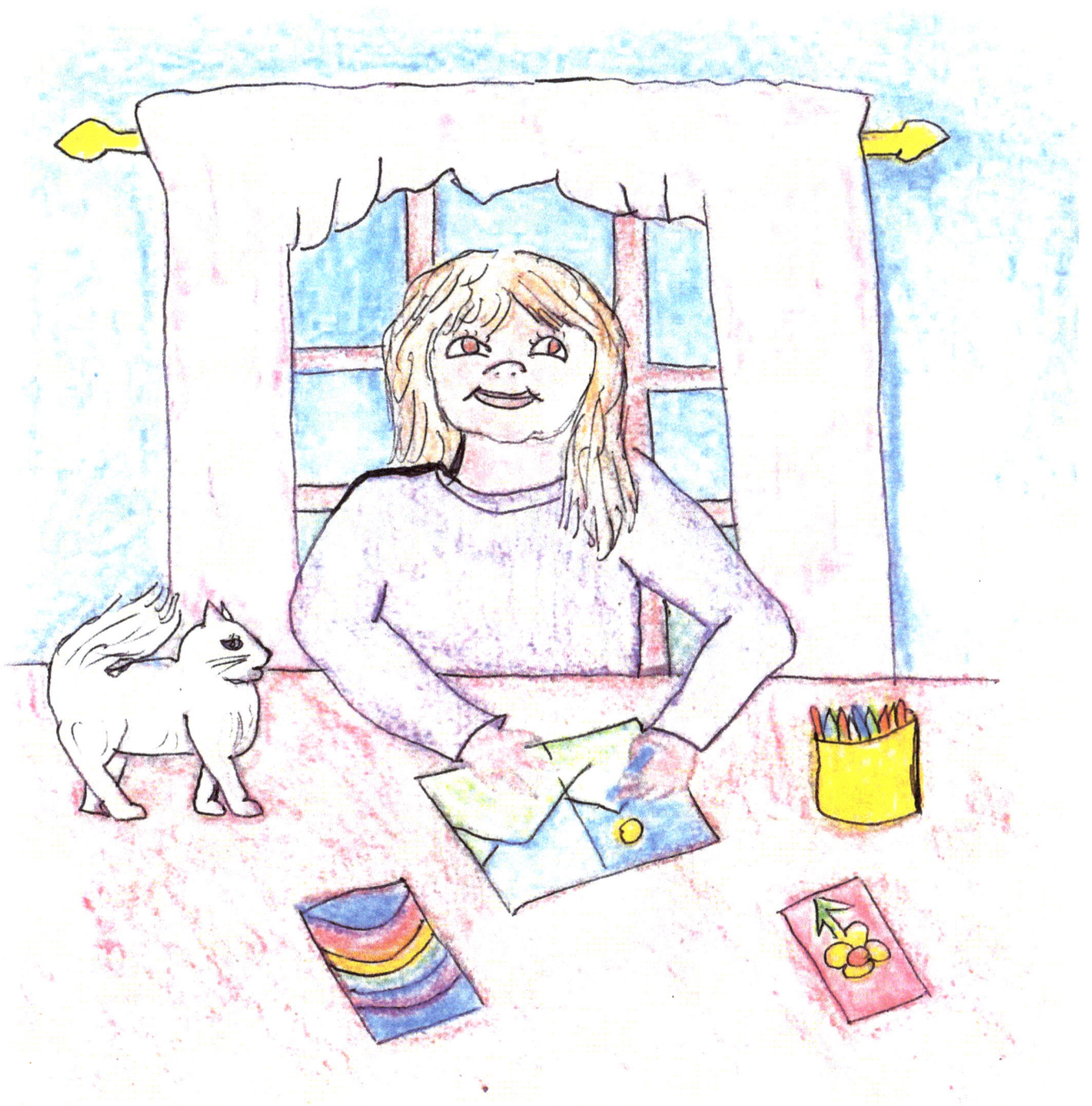

Cc Carol creates colorful cards with her can of crayons.

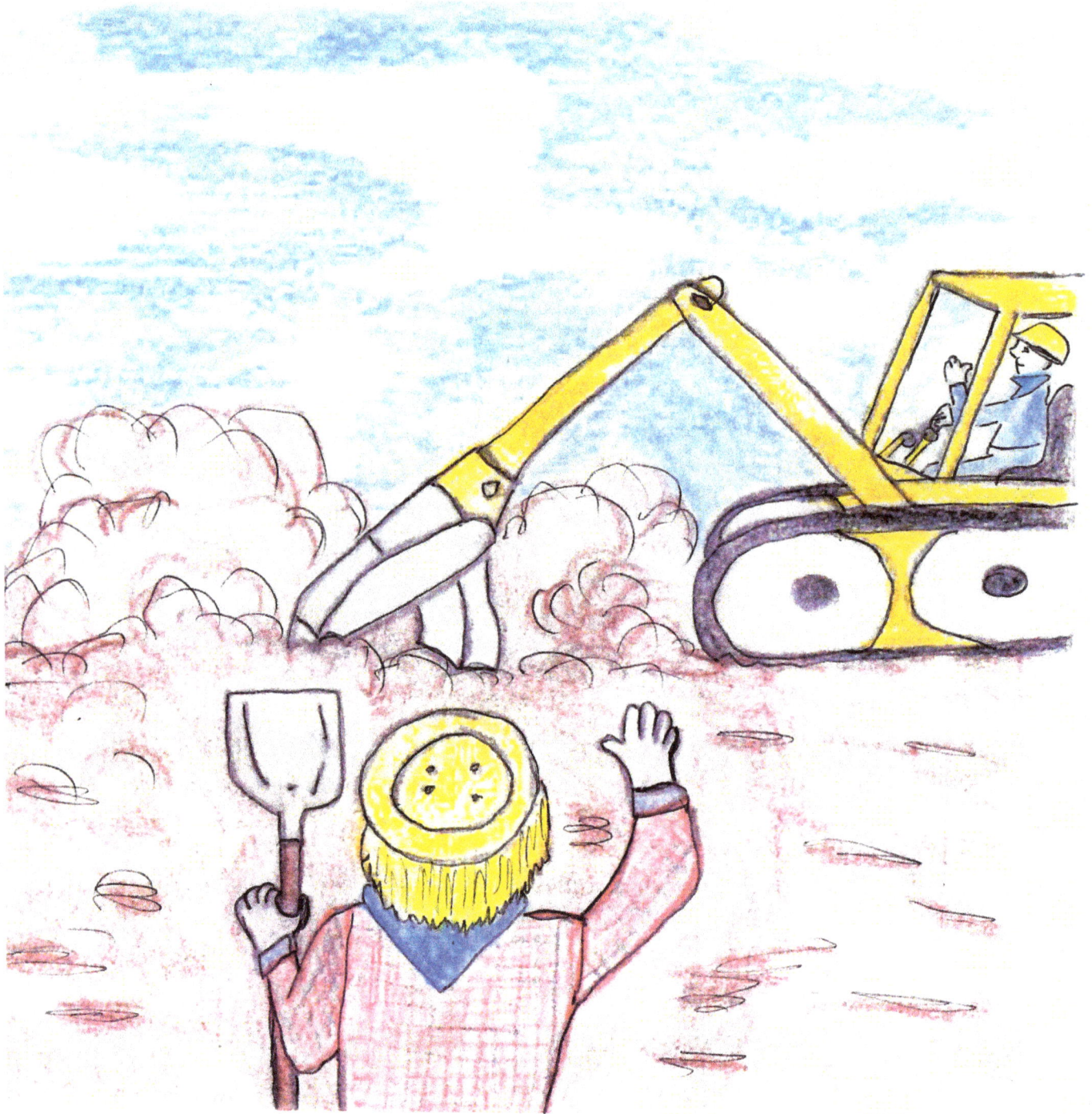

Dd David's dad digs deep ditches in the dusty dirt.

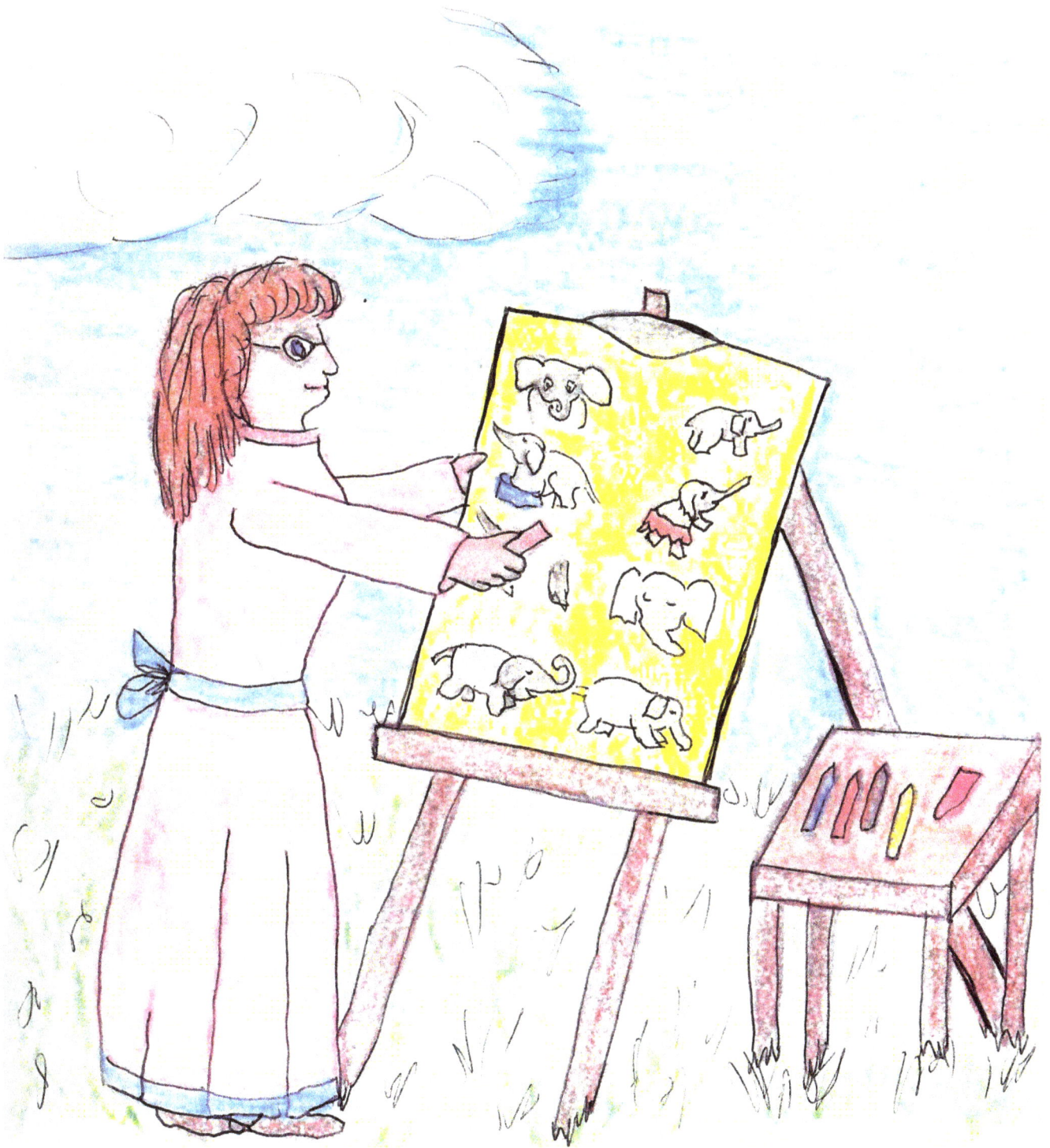

Ee   Ellen erases eight elephants from her easel.

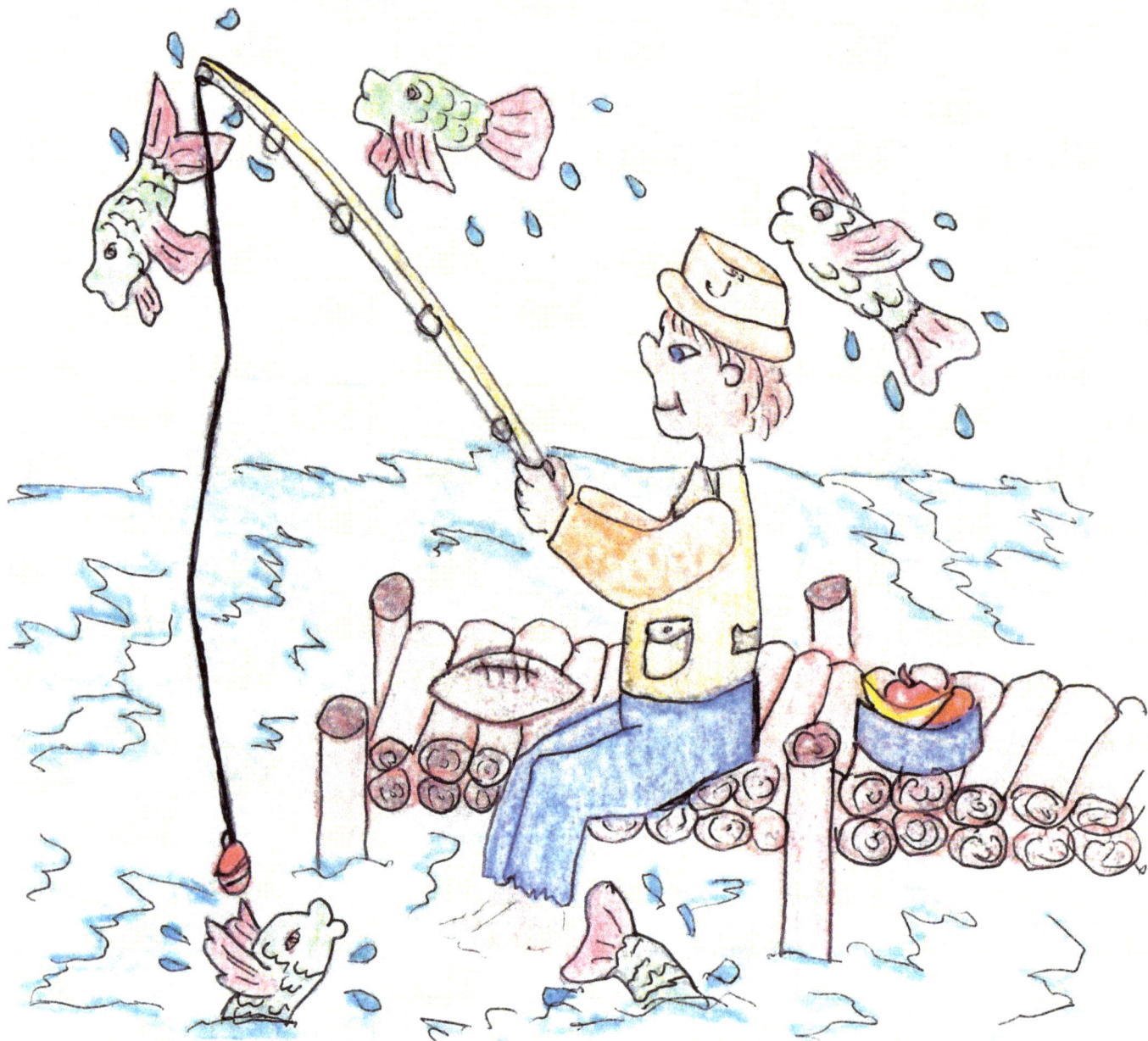

Ff   Frank fishes for five flying fish.

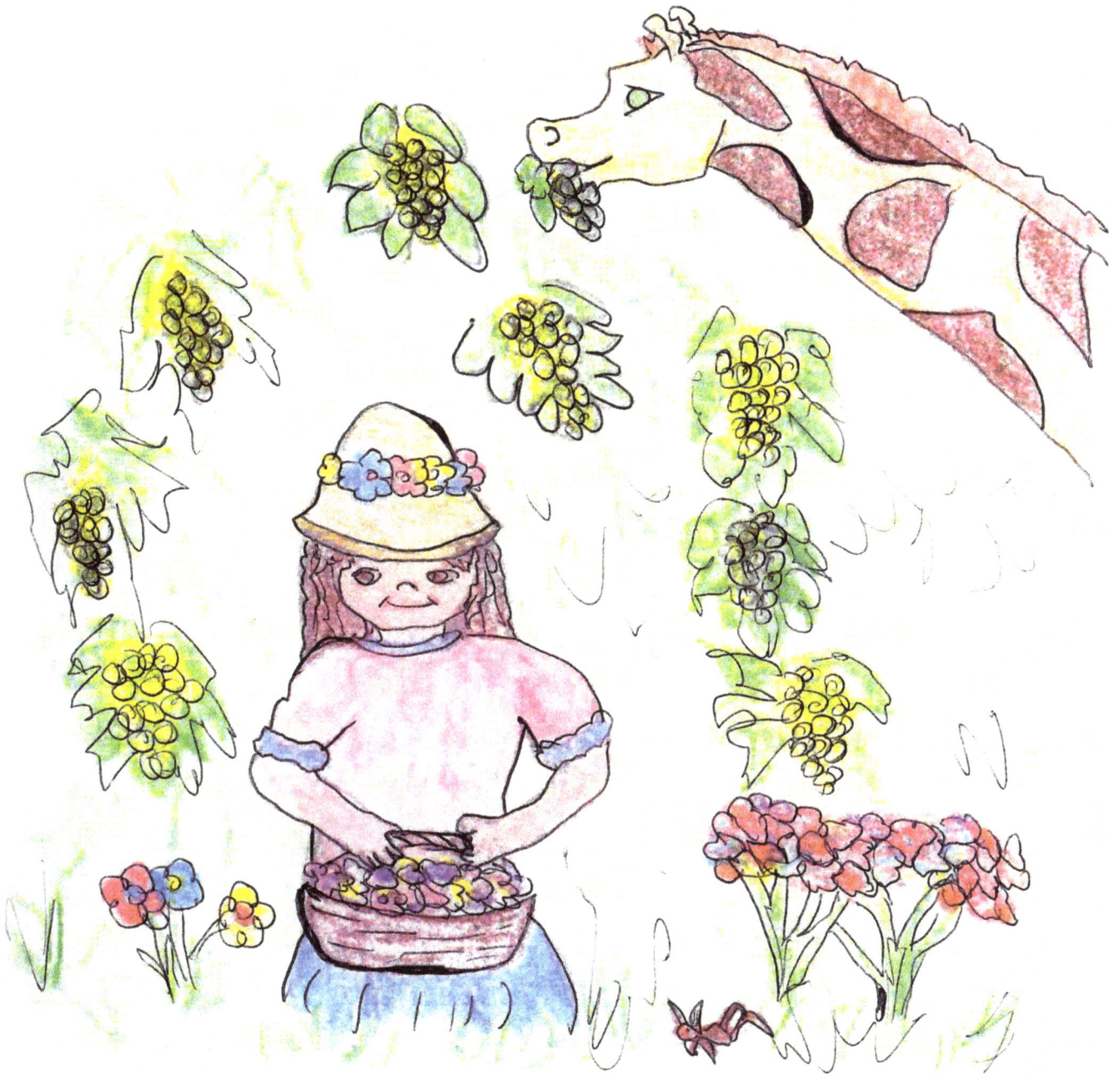

Gg Gail grew green grapes in her gorgeous garden.

Hh

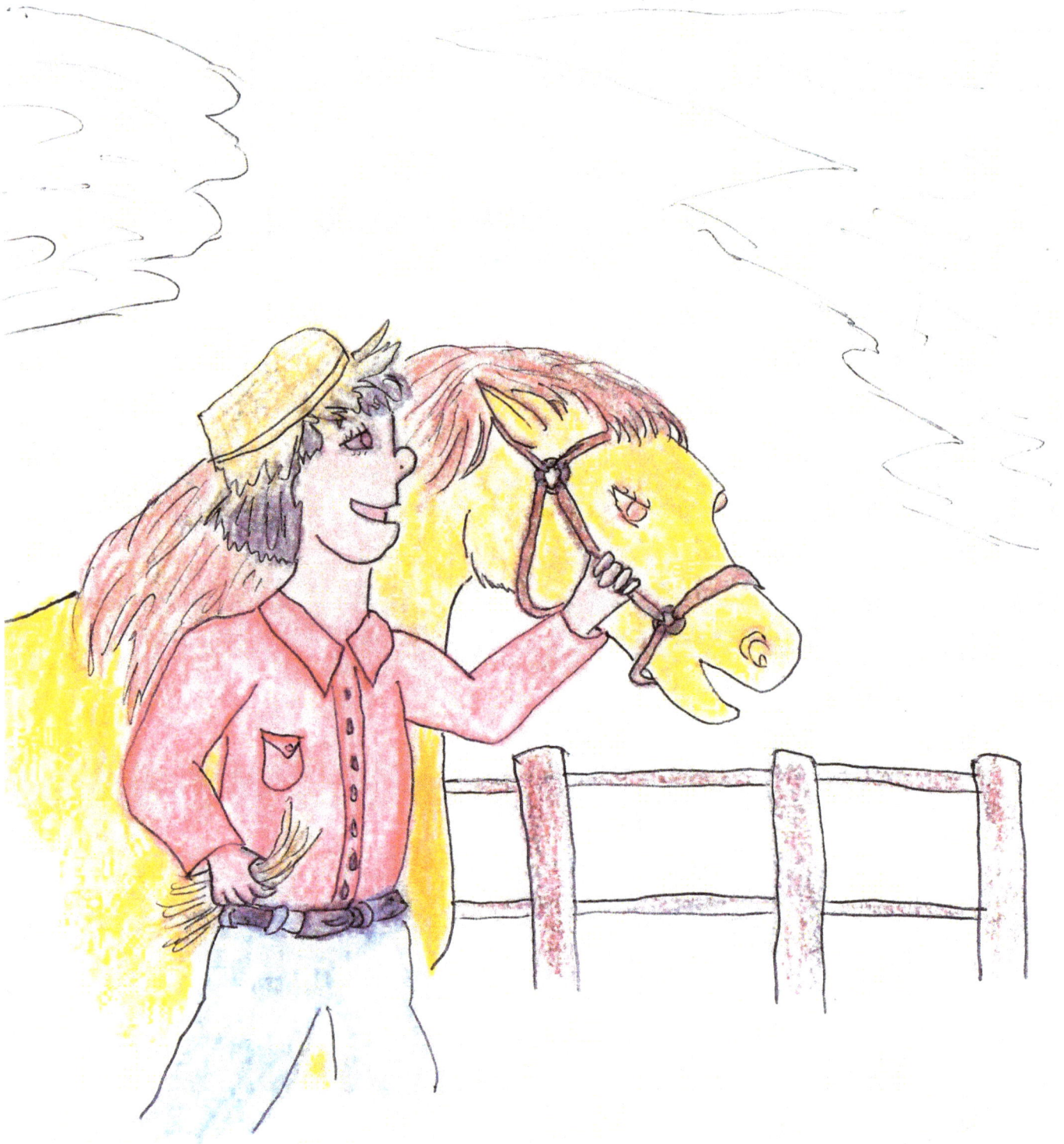

Hank held his horse by her handy halter.

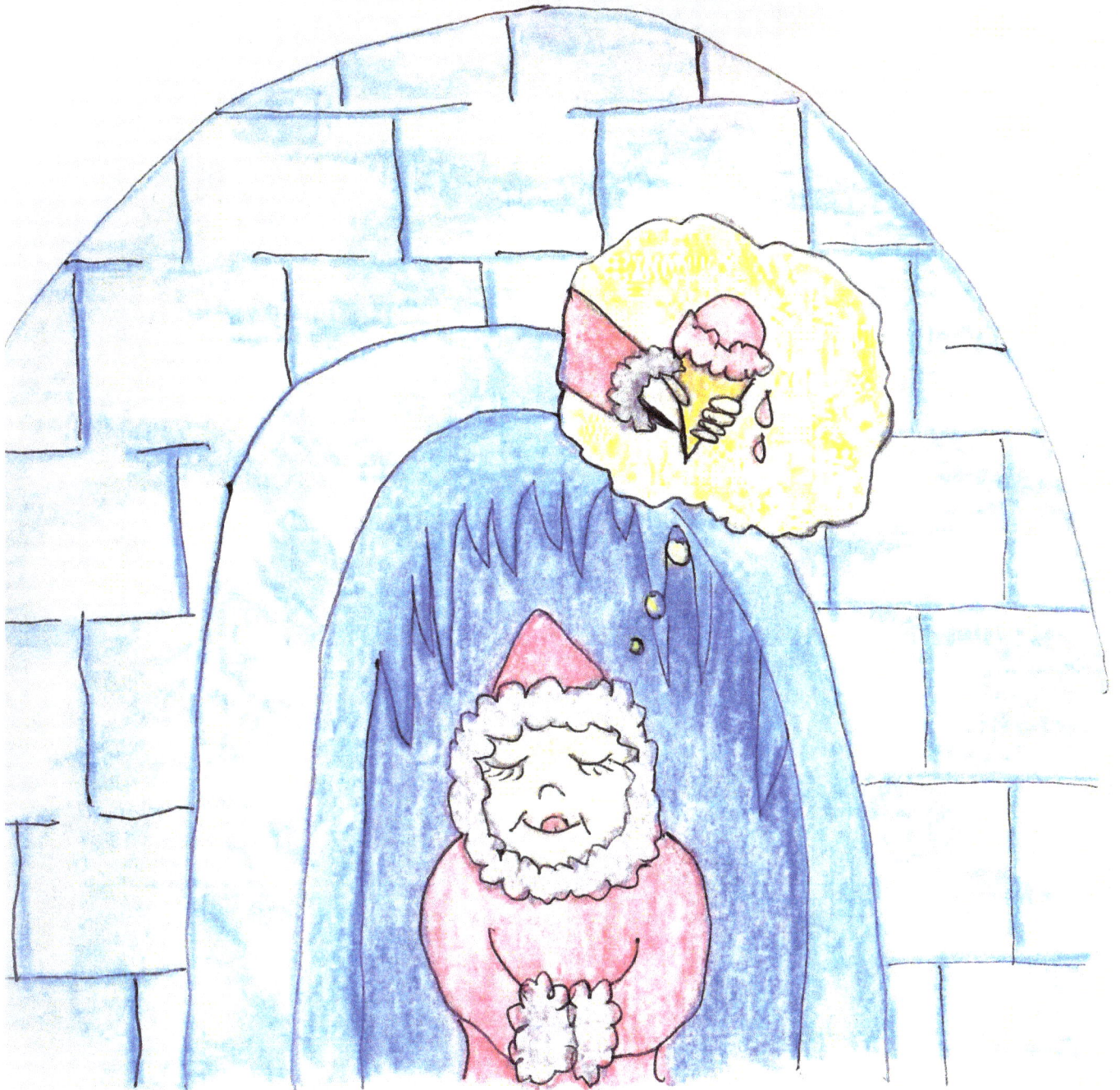

Ii   Ingrid imagined eating her ice cream
while in her icy igloo.

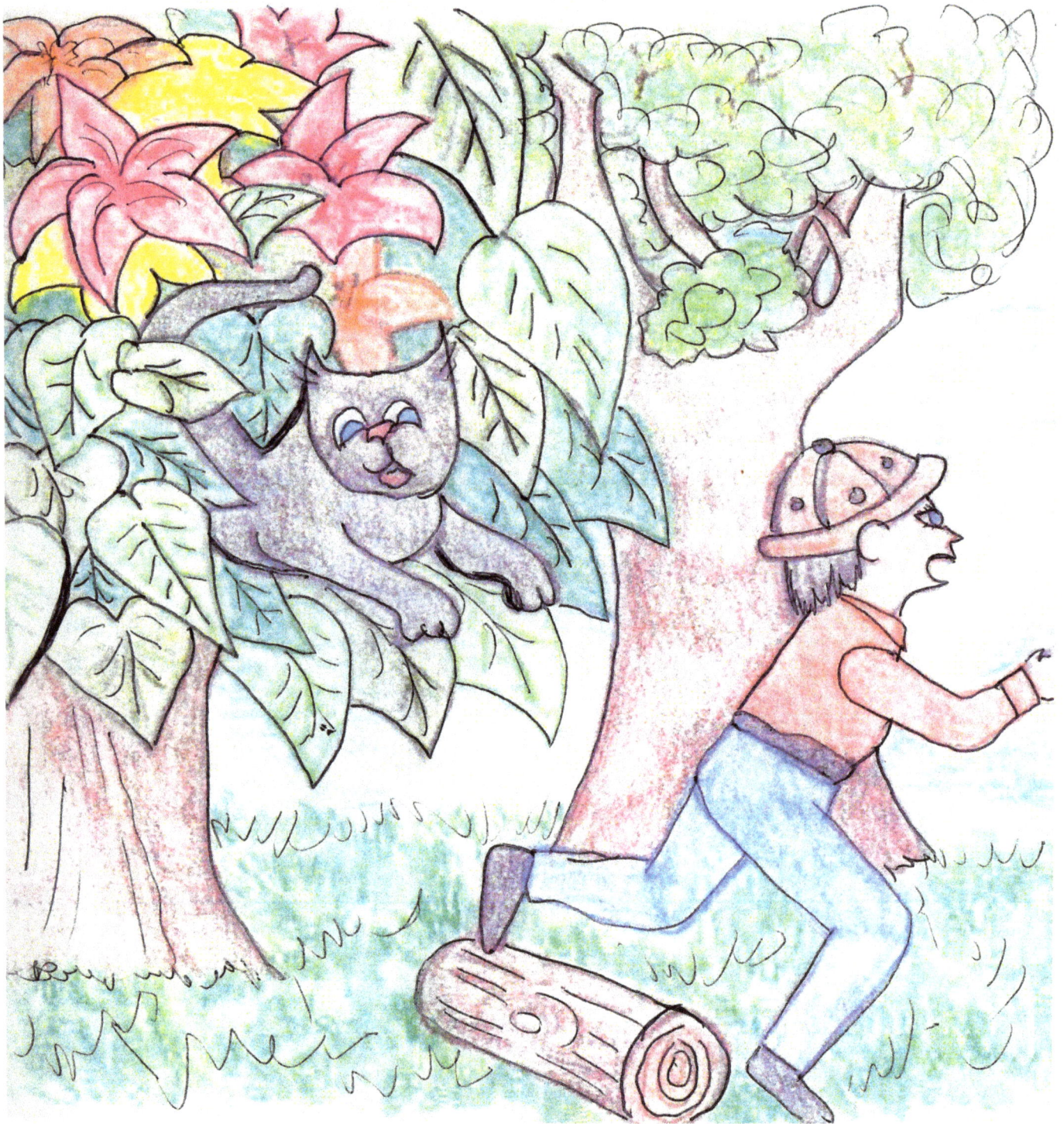

Jj

John jumped when the jaguar jolted from the jungle.

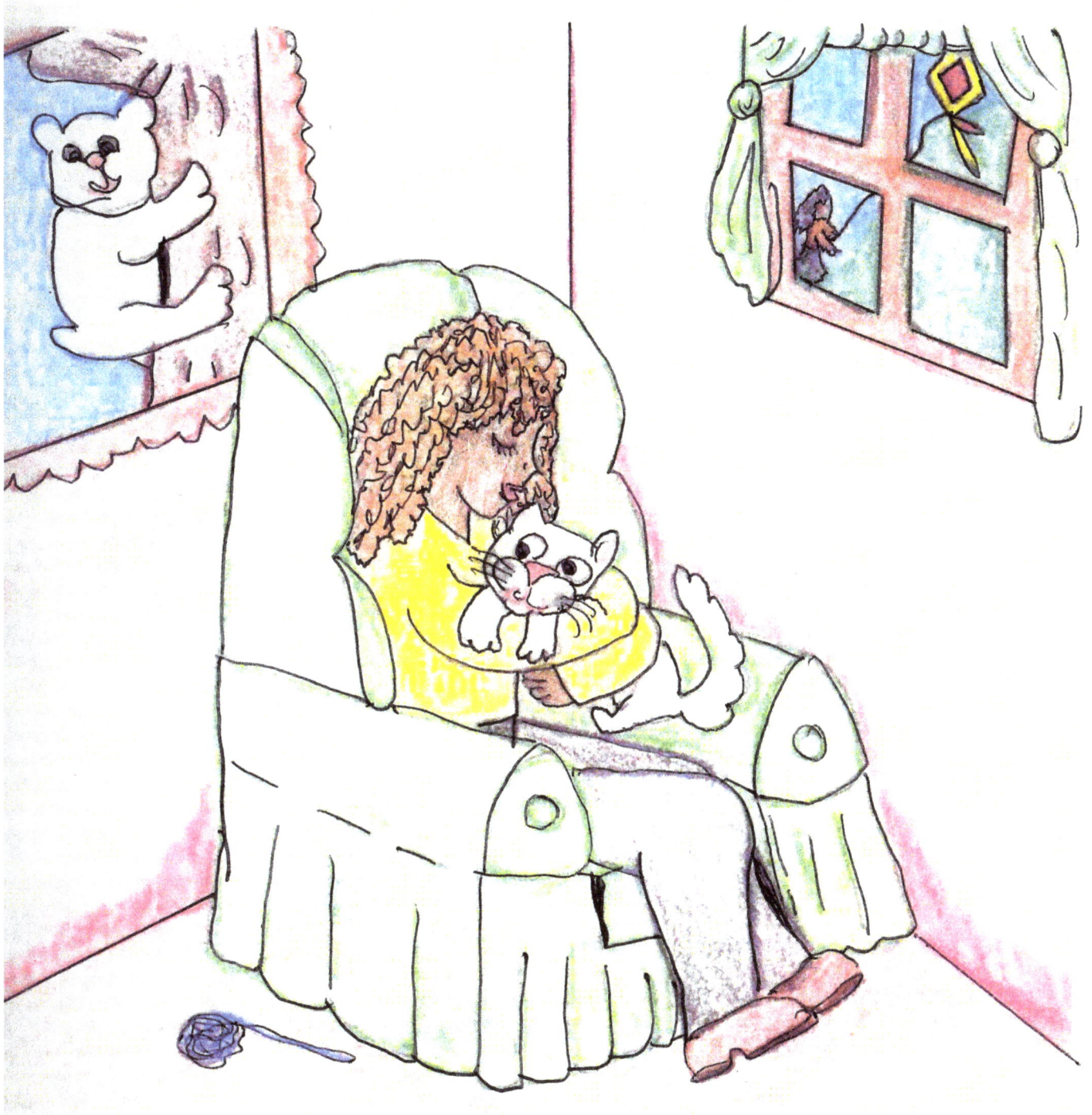

Kk Kate kissed and cuddled her kitten named Koala.

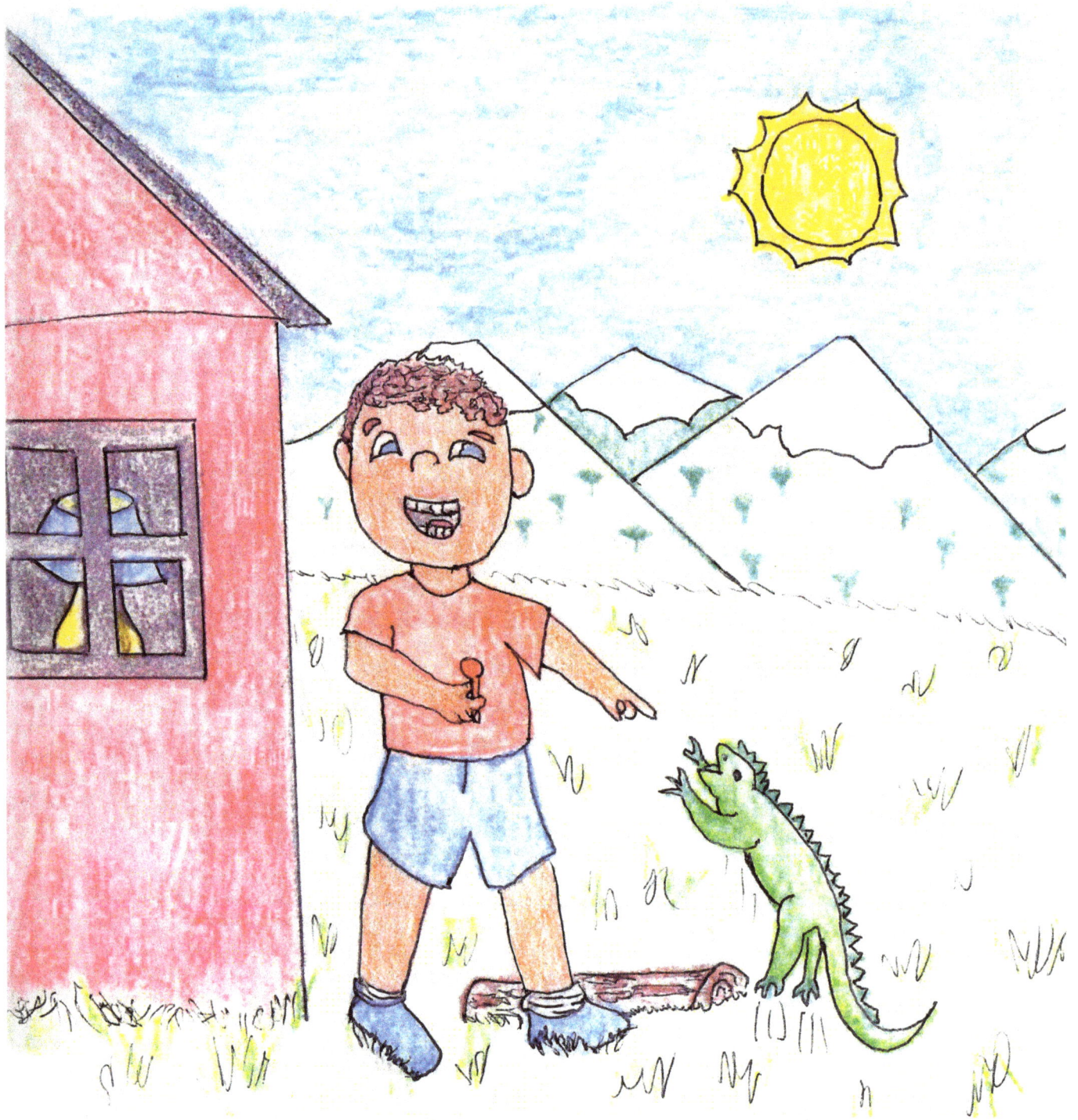

Ll   Larry laughed at Lizzy, his large leaping Lizard.

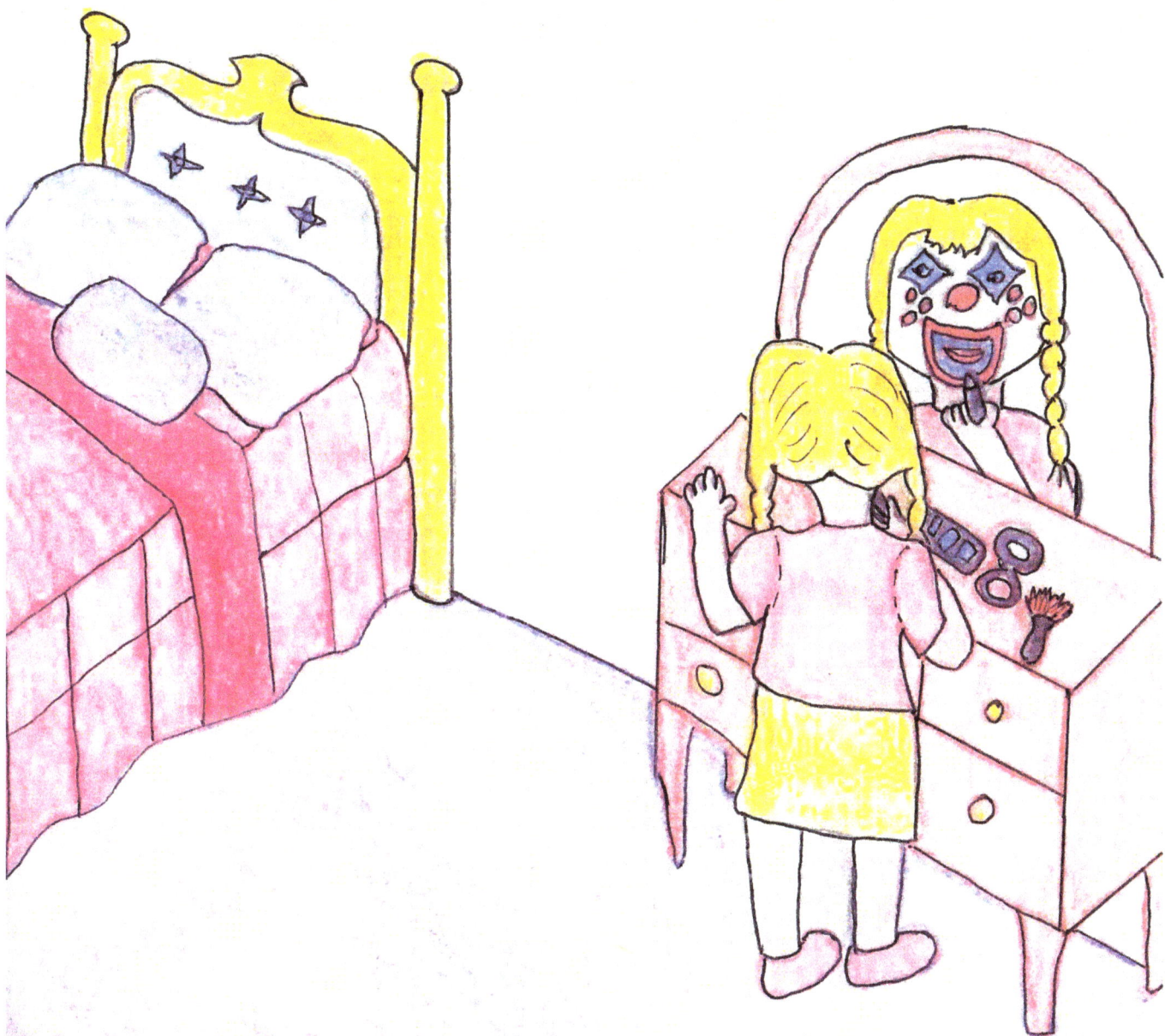

Mm   Margie merrily made a mask with her mom's makeup.

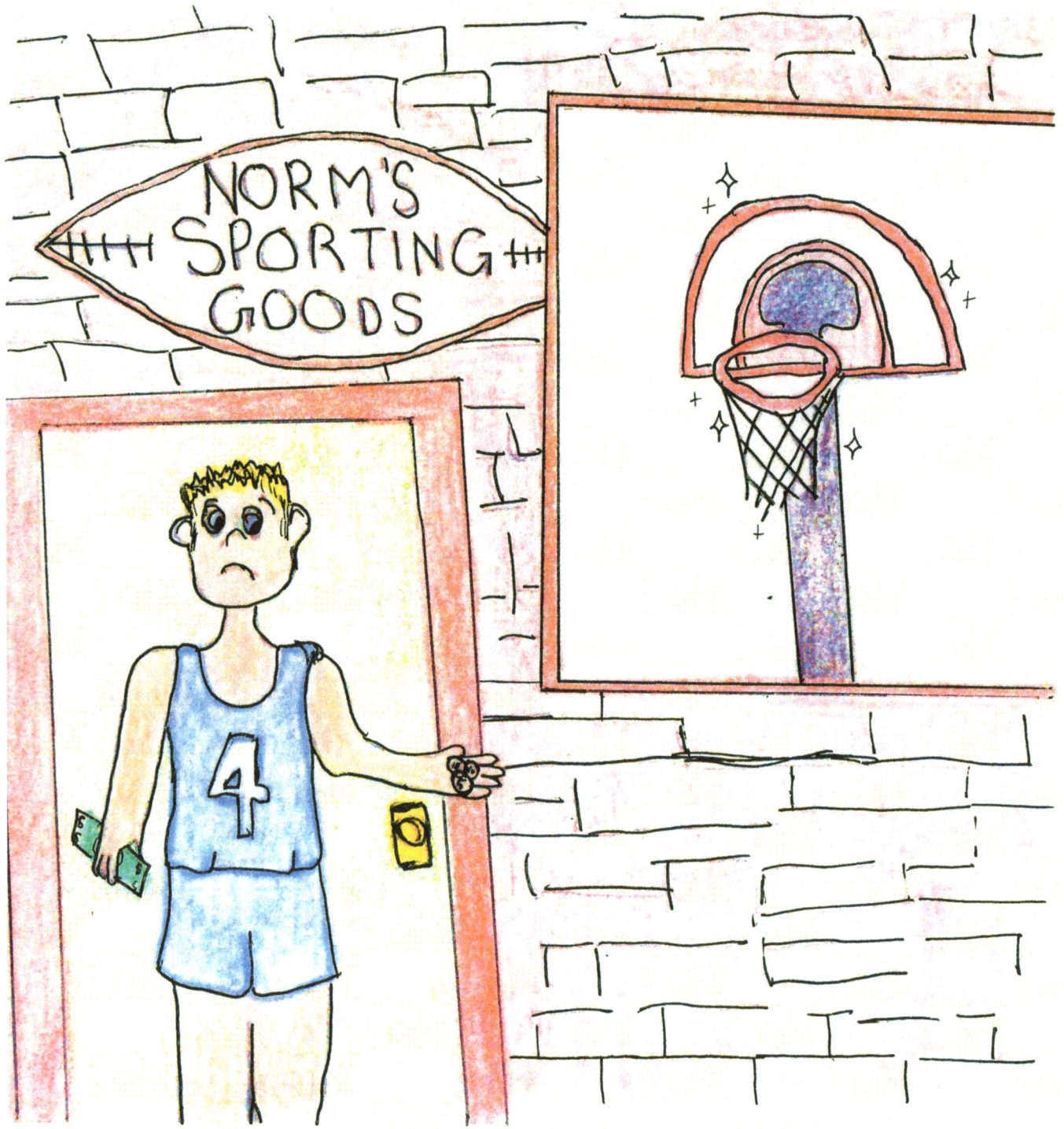

Nn   Nick needed a nickel to buy a new net.

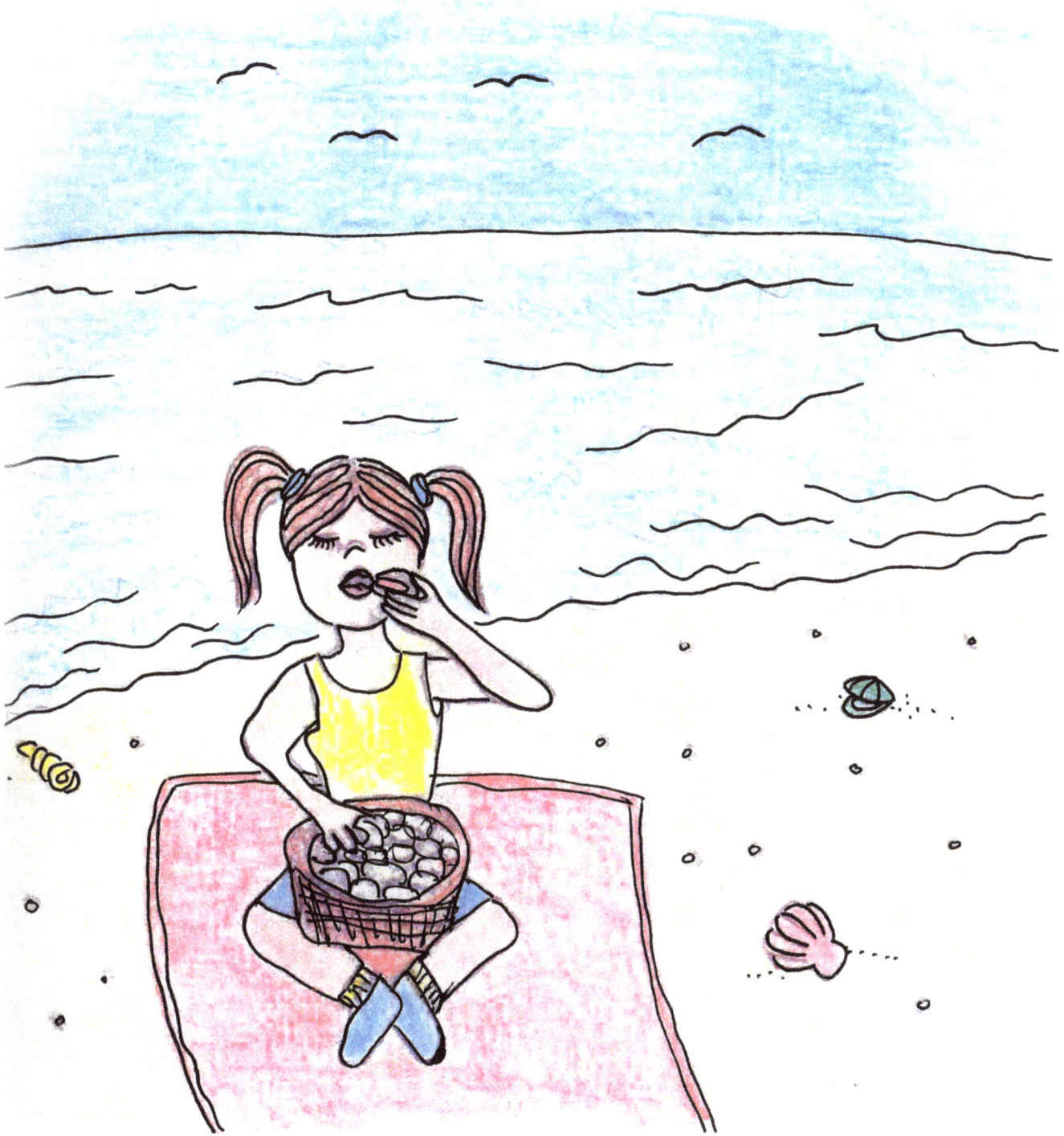

Oo   Odie opened oysters from the ocean and oozed them into her mouth.

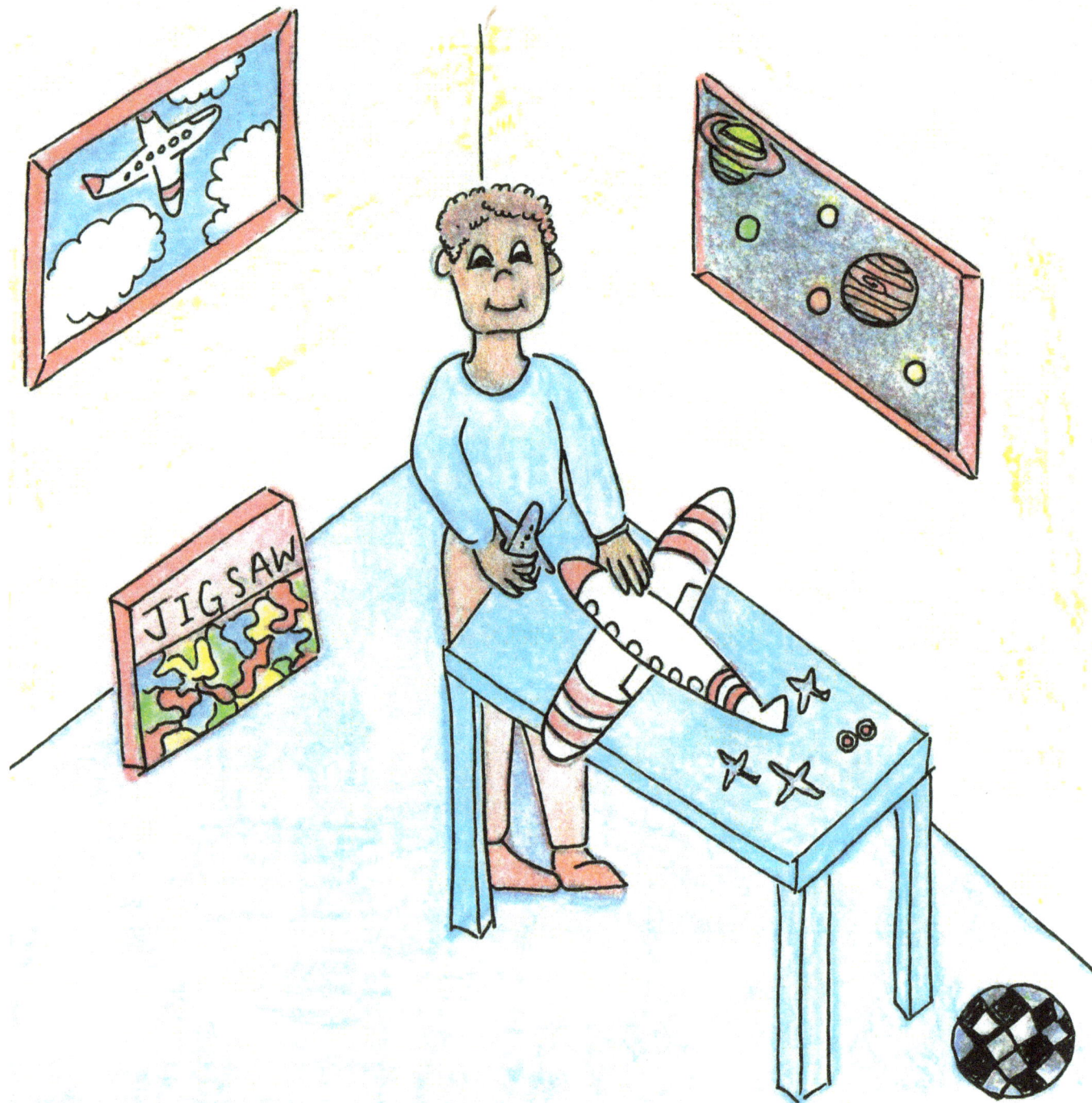

Pp Pete put propellers on his plane while playing in his playroom.

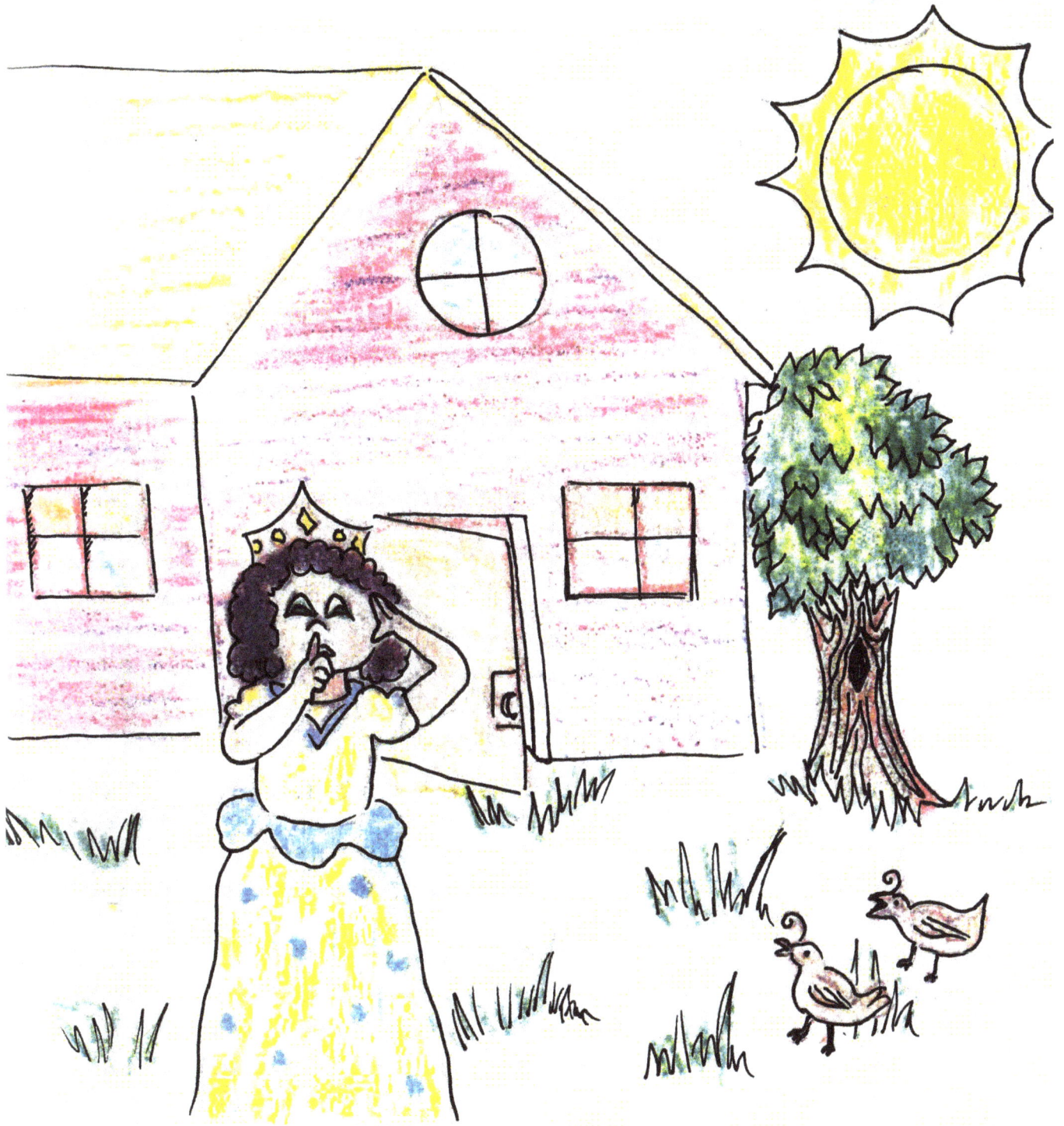

Qq Queenie quietly listened for quirky quacking quails.

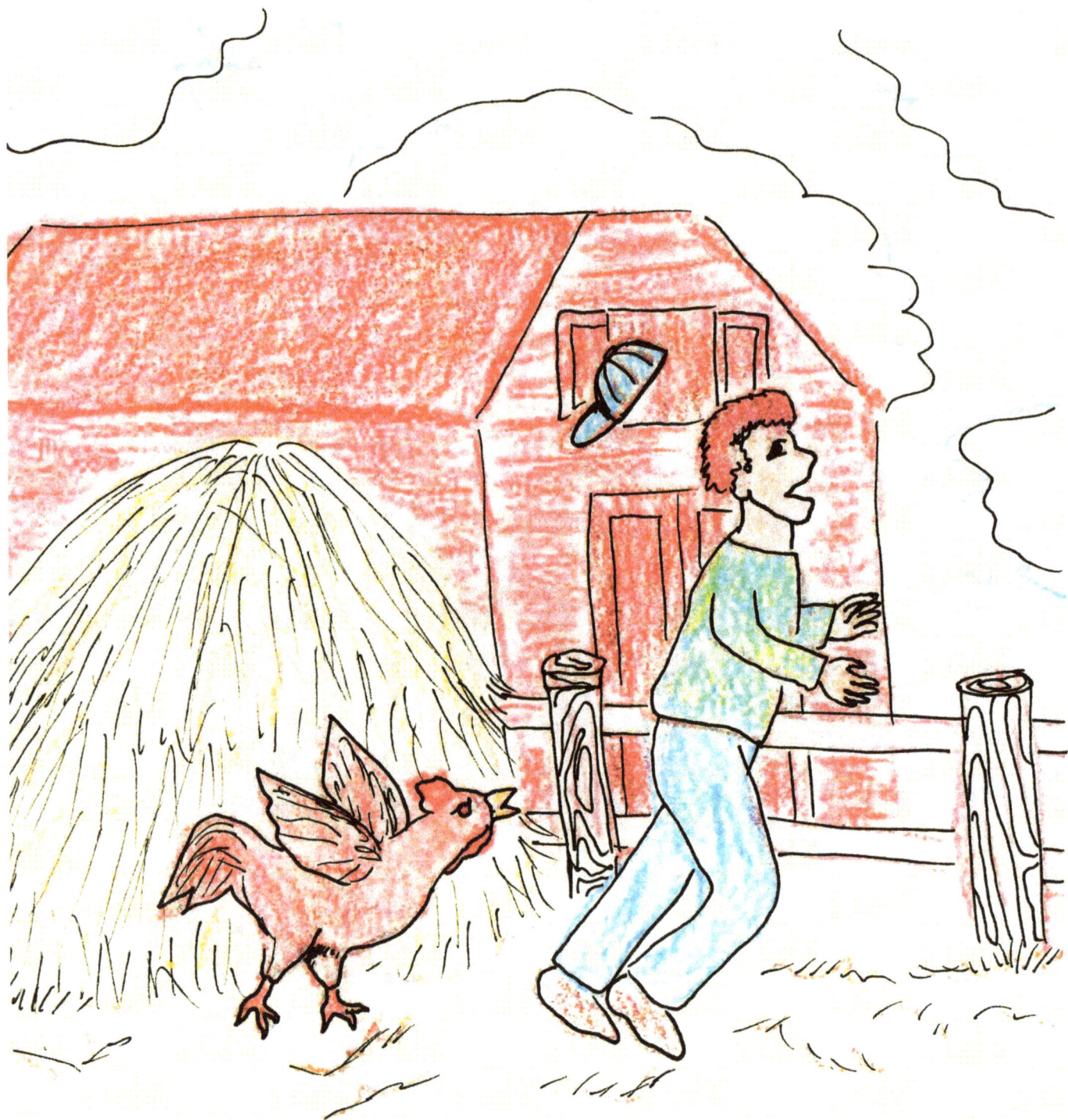

Rr   Ronnie ran rapidly from a rustling
red rooster.

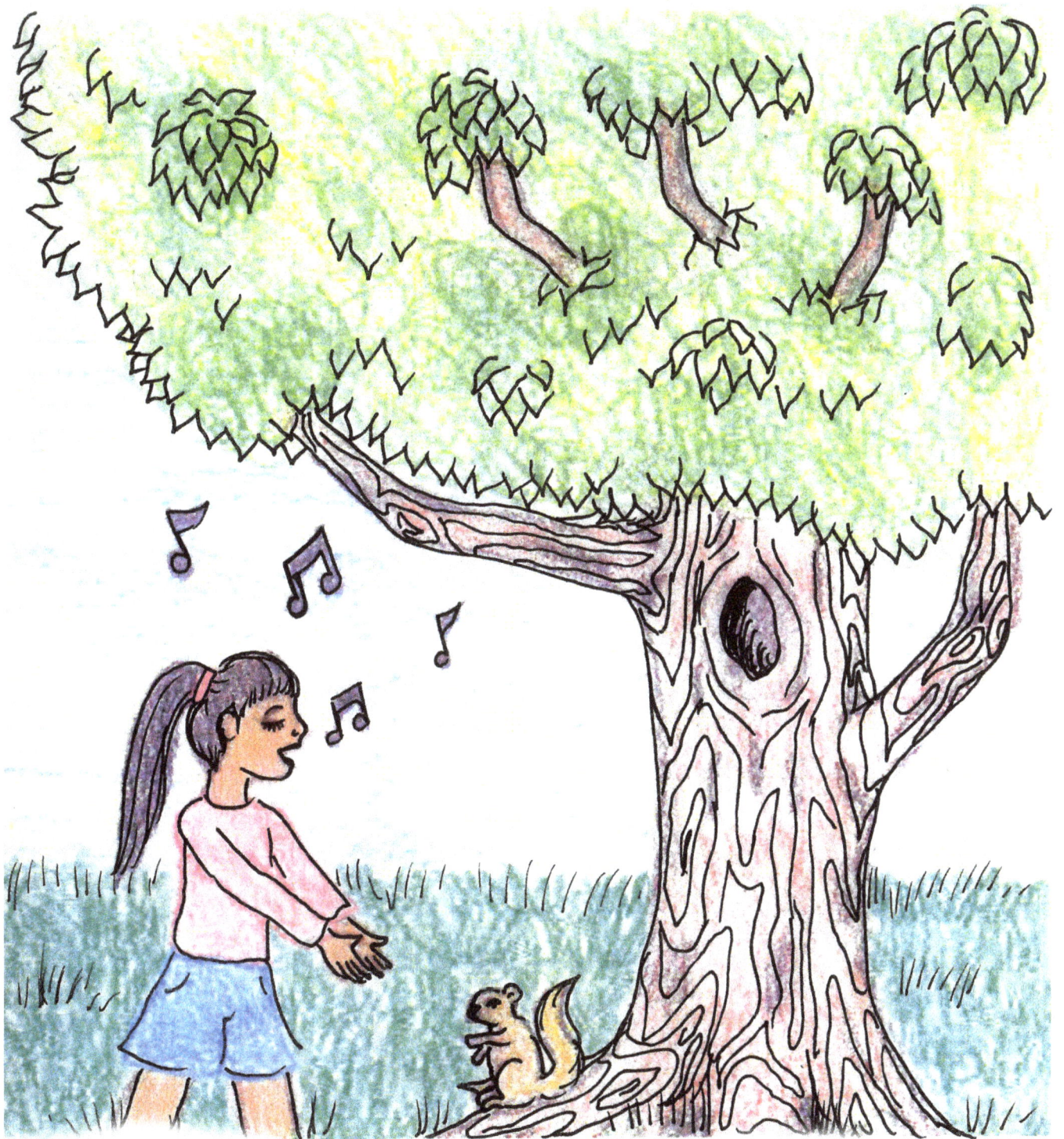

Ss   Sally sang softly to a scared
squiggly squirrel.

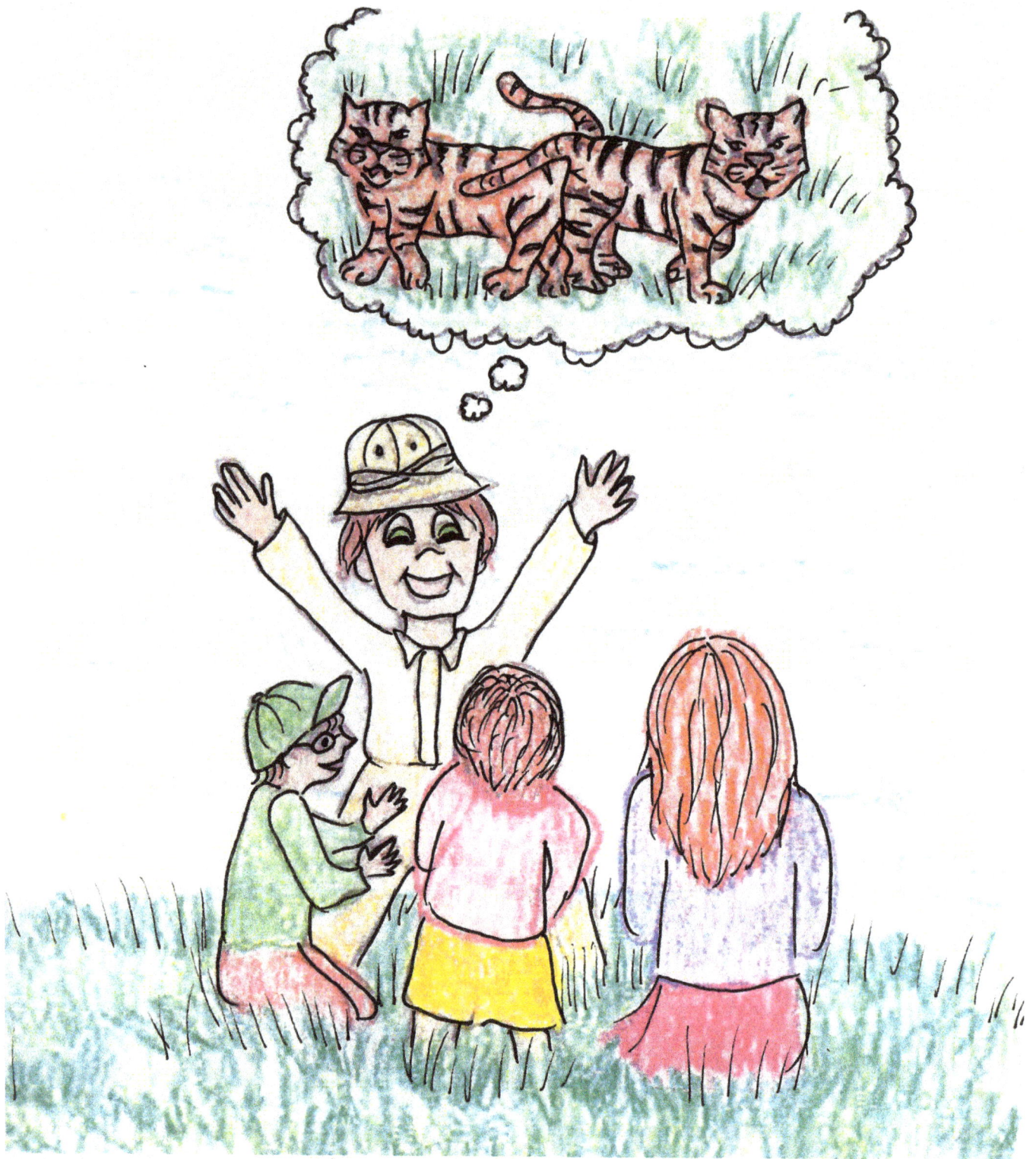

Tt   Todd told tales of tracking two tigers.

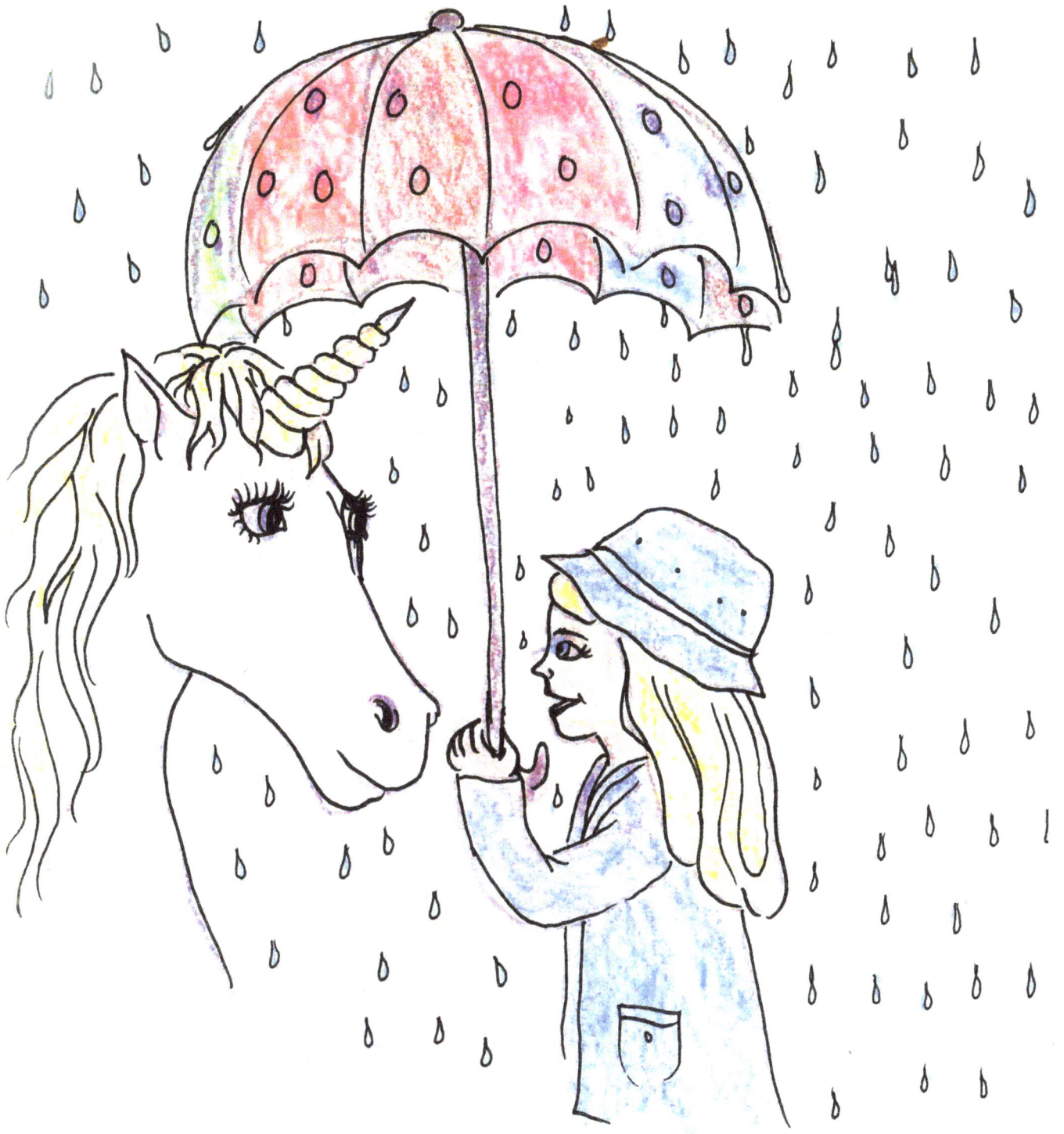

Uu Ursula urged her unicorn under the ugly umbrella.

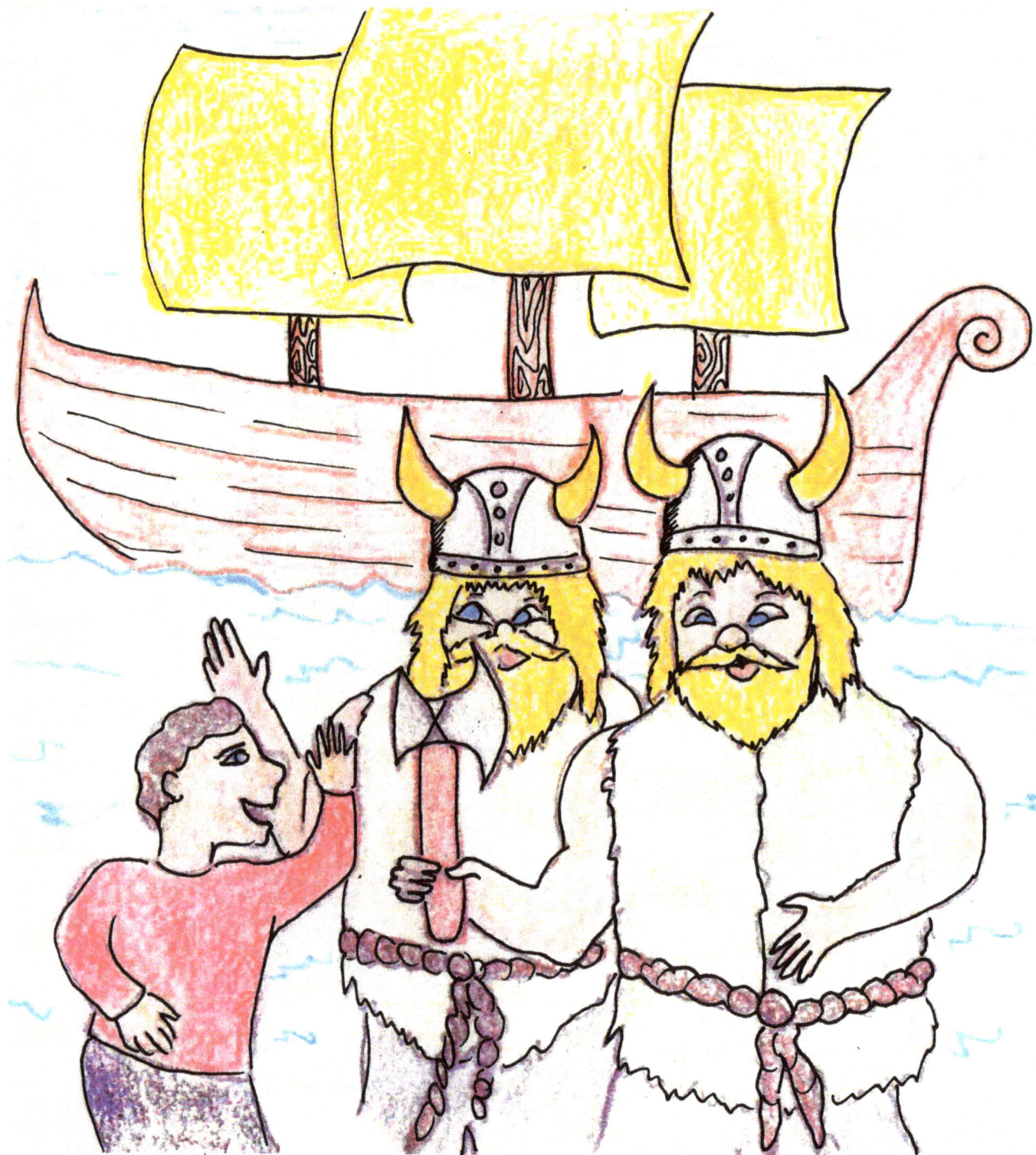

Vv Victor visits with very vicious Vikings.

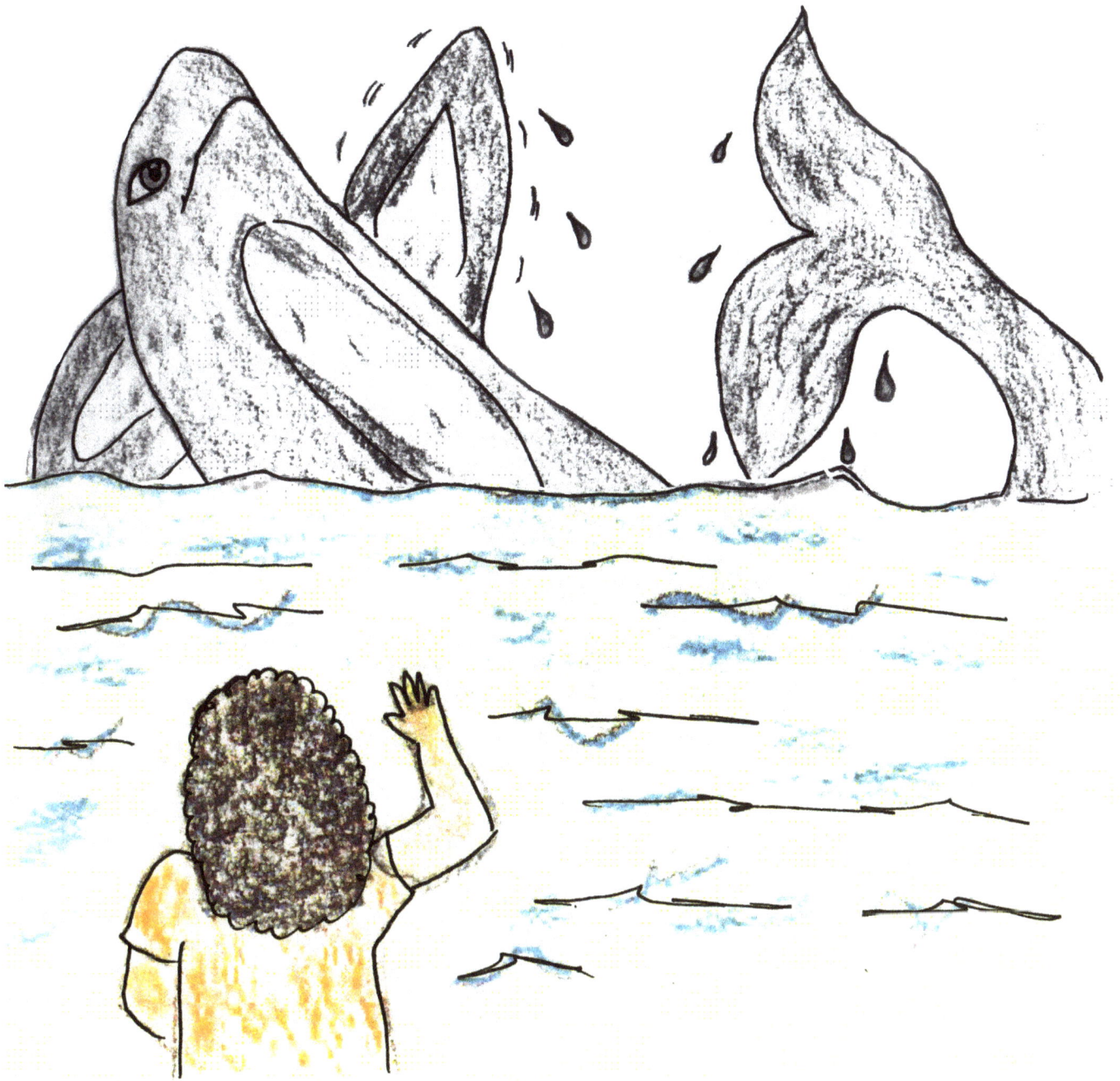

Ww Wendy watches Wally the white
whale waving in the water.

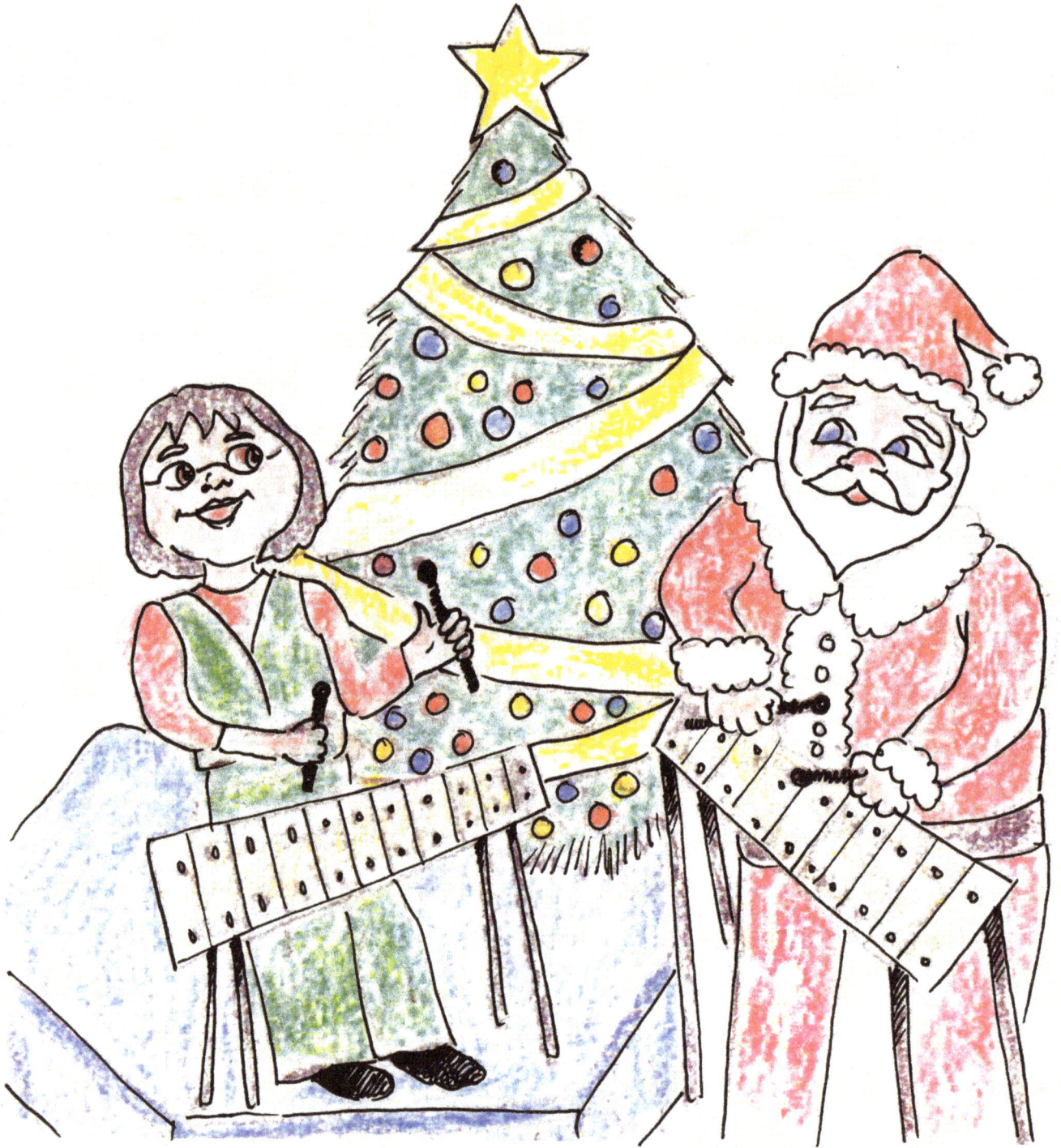

Xx Xavier has extra xylophones to play at Christmas parties.

Yy

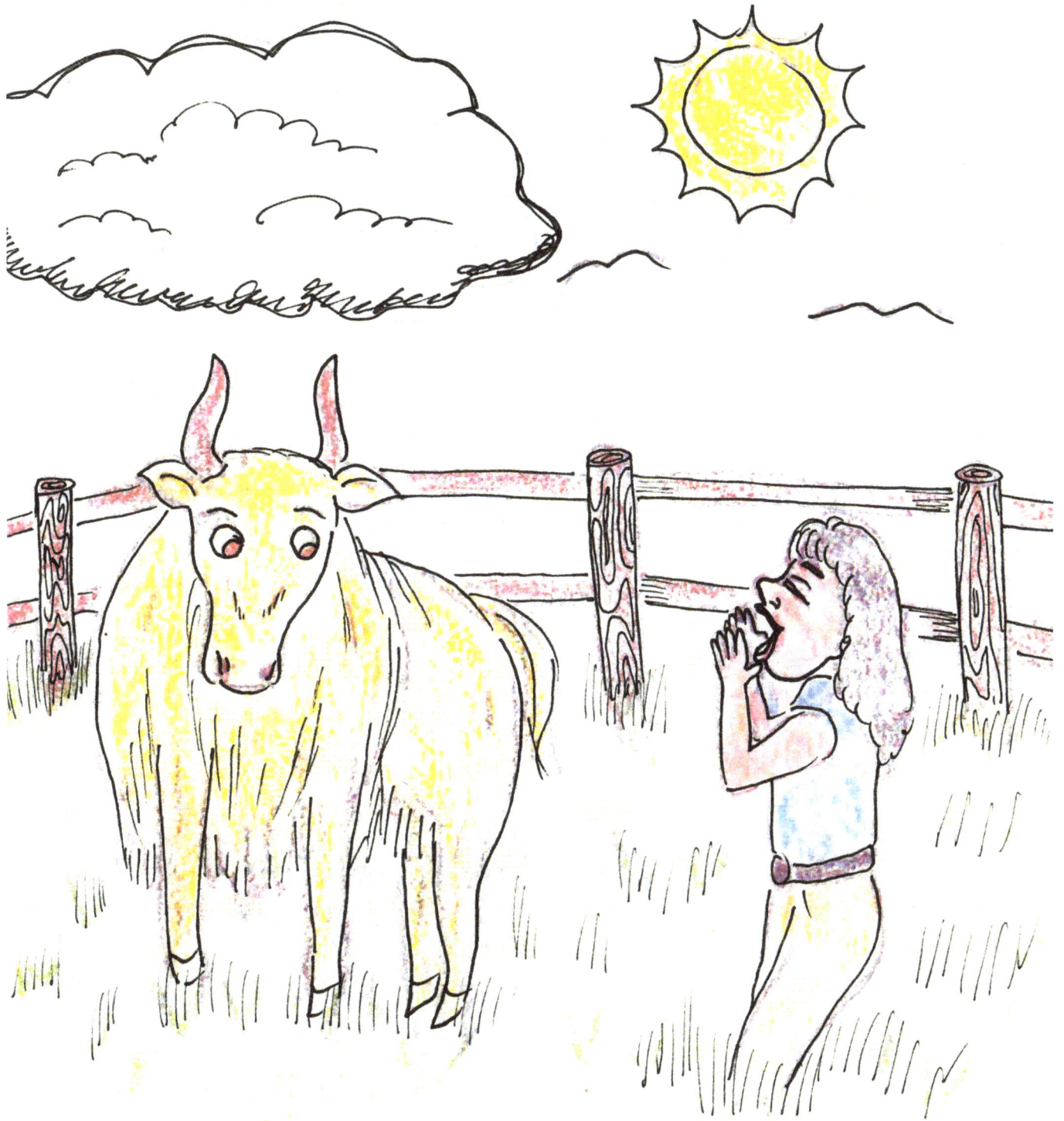

Yolanda yells loudly at the yellow yak.

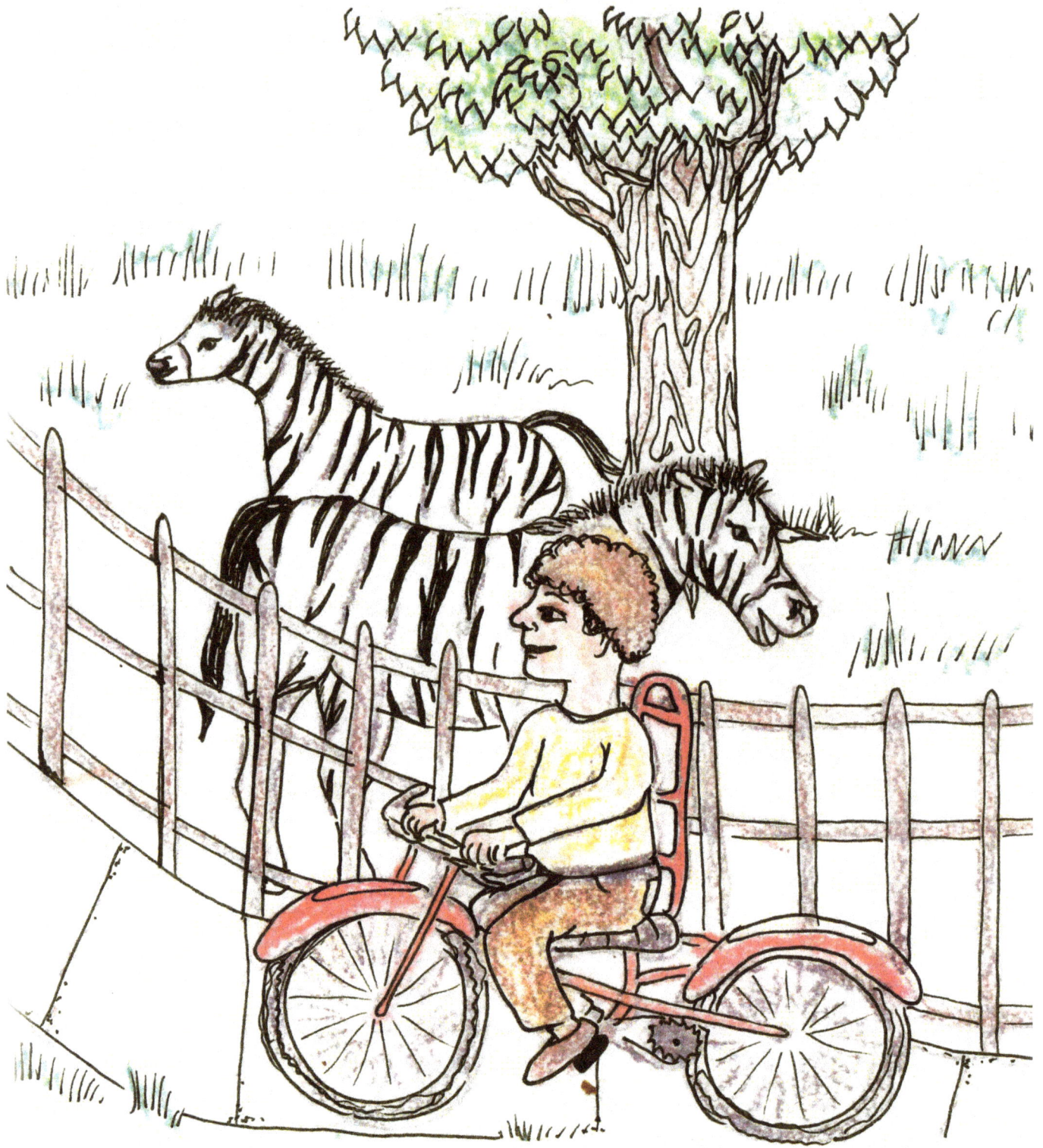

Zz   Zachery zoomed to the zoo to zero in on the zebras.

Comic Sans on LSI 70# archival white
Type and design by Karen Paul Stone

www.ingramcontent.com/pod-product-compliance
Lightning Source LLC
Chambersburg PA
CBHW041604260326

41914CB00011B/1382